Generis
PUBLISHING

THE ROLE OF AUTOHEMOTHERAPY WITH OZONE AS AN EFFECTIVE TREATMENT FOR FIBROMYALGIA

Triantafyllia Dimou

Title: **THE ROLE OF AUTOHEMOTHERAPY WITH OZONE AS AN EFFECTIVE TREATMENT FOR FIBROMYALGIA**

ISBN: 979-8-89966-673-5

Author: Triantafyllia Dimou

Cover image: www.pixabay.com

Publisher: Generis Publishing
Online orders: www.generis-publishing.com
Contact email: info@generis-publishing.com

TABLE OF CONTENTS

Chapter 1: Understanding fibromyalgia

Fibromyalgia is considered to be one of the most frustrating conditions in modern medicine. It has a prevalence of 2 to 4 percent in the general population of the world and a significant preponderance in women, and it is one of the most prevalent causes of chronic pain in clinical practice [1]. However, it is so common that it is often ignored, misdiagnosed or even given to patients as a diagnosis of last resort, when all other explanations have been exhausted.

One of the challenges is that there is no apparent harm on x-rays, no clear abnormality on routine laboratory tests, no lesion which a surgeon can detect or excise. It is a person in considerable and prolonged pain, accompanied by fatigue which sleep fails to relieve, a fog-like mental impairment which patients complain of being unable to think clearly and an assortment of other complaints such as morning stiffness, headaches, gastrointestinal disturbances and an unusual sensitivity to noise, light and temperature. Mood disorders are so prevalent in these patients and especially depression and anxiety that it has come to be viewed as central to the condition and not as a secondary response to being in pain [2]. When put together, it is not the image of a localized injury or infection but rather of a dysregulation that is system wide, a body that has, in some fundamental sense, lost the capacity to regulate its own reactions to the world around it.

The official acceptance of fibromyalgia as a unique medical condition has a not-so-long history, but descriptions of symptom patterns resembling fibromyalgia have been found in the medical literature centuries before that under various names, including fibrositis, muscular rheumatism, and psychogenic rheumatism. Fibromyalgia dates back to the early 1980s, and first widely accepted diagnostic criteria were published by the American College of Rheumatology in 1990. The initial criteria were based on finding tender points, particular areas of the body where patients complained of pain on the application of pressure. They offered a good baseline to begin with, but they were too fixed to a condition as fluctuating and changeable as fibromyalgia. A new set of criteria in 2010 changed the diagnostic focus to a symptom based model, including the Widespread Pain Index and Symptom Severity Scale, and officially considered that fibromyalgia manifests differently in individuals and evolves in character over time [1]. This update was an indicator that fibromyalgia was now beginning to be accepted more by the medical community.

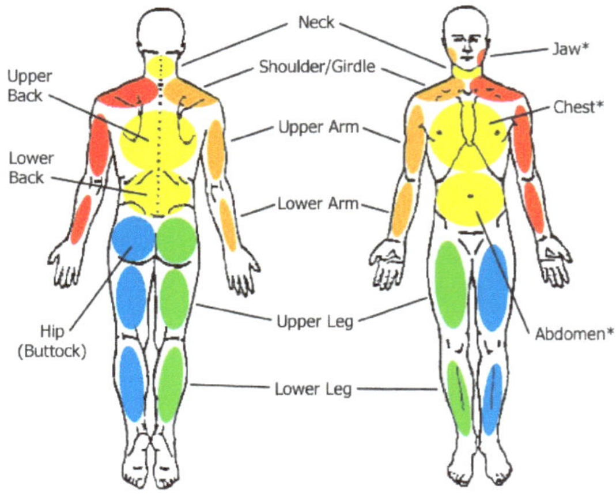

Figure 1. *Widespread pain areas in fibromyalgia [3].*

To the patients, though, the rate of change in clinical practice has been significantly slower than the rate of scientific knowledge. Average delays between symptom onset and a confirmed diagnosis have always been recorded at five to seven years. In the process, at that time, patients are shuffled among various specialists, they have repeated and unnecessary tests and treatments that are directed at the wrong conditions. The physical, psychological and financial cost of this trip is immense. Recent studies have been undertaken to find biological indicators, which may reduce this time of diagnostic delay and provide more confidence, but none of the indicators have so far been accurate enough to be used consistently in clinical practice [4]. What it does not imply by this lack is that fibromyalgia does not have a biological basis.

The sensitized nervous system

The central sensitization concept is the last contribution of recent neuroscience to fibromyalgia. Pain is a signal in a healthy nervous system that is proportionate to the stimulus that causes it. In fibromyalgia, such proportionality fails in a very particular manner. The central nervous system becomes sensitive to exaggerate its responses, and interprets normal sensory data like it is dangerous and responds to actually painful stimuli with a level of intensity much greater than would be justified by tissue damage in the periphery alone. A touch of light is painful and even slight fluctuation of temperature results in discomfort. The body, in this condition, is reacting in a true change in how the nervous system of its own has been tuned [5].

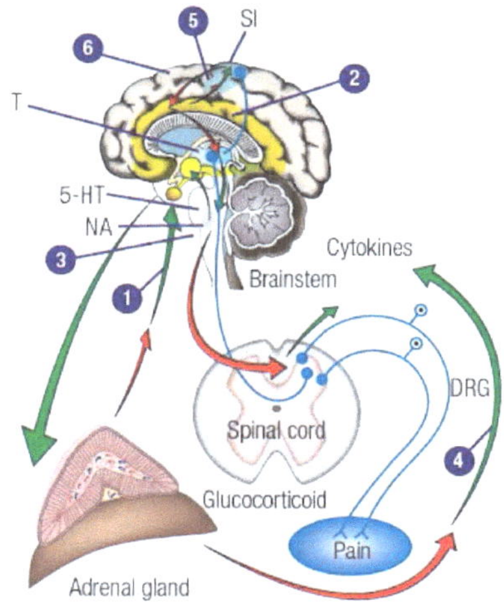

Figure 2. *Schematic of descending disinhibition and central pain sensitization pathways [6].*

Oxidative stress and the biology of chronic pain

Amongst the more disclosing findings in fibromyalgia research has been the consistent occurrence of increased oxidative stress in patients with the disorder, which has been found to be strong across various independent studies. Oxidative stress occurs when the generation of reactive oxygen species surpasses the ability of the antioxidant defense systems in the body, causing cellular and molecular damage. Lipid peroxidation products, protein oxidation indicators, and antioxidant enzyme activity measurements in fibromyalgia patients are significantly different to those of healthy individuals [7]. They follow closely clinical severity and usually the level of oxidative damage is higher in patients who complain of more pain. The lived experience and the biological signal are either on the same track, which implies that oxidative stress does not result in the condition but is an active part of its pathology [8].

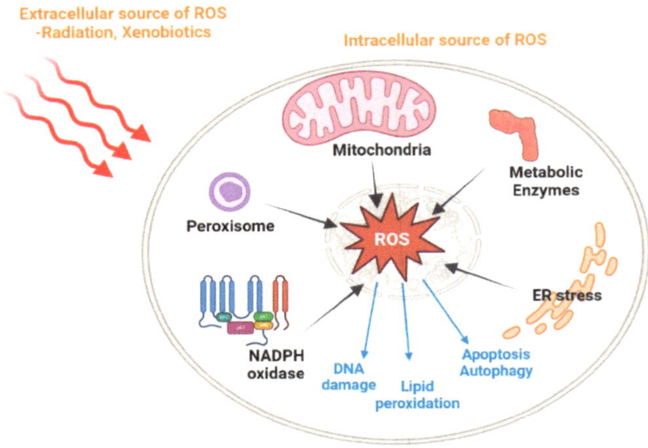

***Figure 3**. Oxidative stress caused by intracellular and extracellular stimuli schematically depicted. The production of reactive oxygen species primarily occurs in mitochondria, peroxisome and endoplasmic reticulum, and enzymes of metabolism. Over-production results in apoptosis, autophagy, lipid peroxidation, and DNA damage [9].*

Recent studies have verified that these markers have significant diagnostic implications and that the association between them and fibromyalgia is also applicable in the psychological levels including anxiety and depression [10]. Reactive oxygen and nitrogen species interact with ion channels and nociceptive neurons altering the same signaling pathways that have already been perturbed by central sensitization [11]. An additional layer to this scene is mitochondrial dysfunction that produces an excessive production of reactive oxygen species as a by-product of the broken energy metabolism, and might contribute to the depth of fatigue and muscle-related symptoms that patients with fibromyalgia constantly complain of. It has also been shown that the predisposition to these oxidative disturbances is, at least partially, genetic and differences in antioxidant regulatory genes affect those individuals biologically more susceptible to developing the condition [12].

Out of all this comes a situation where the nervous system, the immune system, and metabolic environment has become dys-regulated in a mutually supporting fashion. Central sensitization increases pain, and oxidative stress enhances neural excitability and adds to cellular damage. Both processes are aggravated by poor sleep. In addition, malnutrition and intestinal microbiota imbalances exert further stress on a system already underperforming in terms of keeping the balance in check [13]. None of the elements in this network bears the full load of the disease, and none of the interventions designed to target one of them will provide the type of long-term improvement that patients require and this is the main problem of fibromyalgia. It is worth exploring what has actually been achieved by current treatment and where, regardless of decades of clinical practice, they still fall short before getting to the question of what might work better.

References

1. Gyorfi M, Rupp A, Abd-Elsayed A. Fibromyalgia pathophysiology. Biomedicines. 2022 Nov 29;10(12):3070.

2. Jones EA, Asaad F, Patel N, Jain E, Abd-Elsayed A. Management of fibromyalgia: an update. Biomedicines. 2024 Jun 6;12(6):1266.

3. American Fibromyalgia Syndrome Association (AFSA). Fibromyalgia diagnosis [Internet]. Available from: www.fibromyalgiafund.org/diagnosis/

4. Smeets Y, Soer R, Chatziantoniou E, Preuper RH, Reneman MF, Wolff AP, Timmerman H. Role of non-invasive objective markers for the rehabilitative diagnosis of central sensitization in patients with fibromyalgia: a systematic review. Journal of Back and Musculoskeletal Rehabilitation. 2024 May;37(3):525-84.

5. Hladkykh FV, Liadova TI, Matvieienko MS, Komorovsky R, Smiyan S, Student V. Central sensitization and nociplastic pain: shared mechanisms in fibromyalgia, osteoarthritis, and inflammatory arthritis. Journal of Pain Research. 2026 Dec 31:571311.

6. Roberts A, Lorduy K, Gatchel RJ. Central sensitization: Common etiology in somatoform disorders. Practical Pain Management. 2013;13(2):46-55.

7. Chung CP, Titova D, Oeser A, Randels M, Avalos I, Milne GL, Morrow JD, Stein CM. Oxidative stress in fibromyalgia and its relationship to symptoms. Clinical Rheumatology. 2009 Apr;28(4):435-8.

8. Assavarittirong C, Samborski W, Grygiel-Gorniak B. Oxidative stress in fibromyalgia: from pathology to treatment. Oxidative Medicine and Cellular Longevity. 2022;2022(1):1582432.

9. Hong Y, Boiti A, Vallone D, Foulkes NS. Reactive oxygen species signaling and oxidative stress: transcriptional regulation and evolution. Antioxidants. 2024 Mar 1;13(3):312.

10. Uslu EY, Uslu MF, Yildiz S, Tabara MF. Evaluating oxidative stress in fibromyalgia: diagnostic utility and its relationship with clinical and psychological parameters. Medicina. 2025 Jul 10;61(7):1248.

11. Ho T, Ryan M, Holle J. Redox reactions in chronic pain: mechanisms and relevance in fibromyalgia. Frontiers in Pain Research. 2025 May 13;6:1593908.

12. Rus A, Robles-Fernandez I, Martinez-Gonzalez LJ, Carmona R, Alvarez-Cubero MJ. Influence of oxidative stress-related genes on susceptibility to fibromyalgia. Nursing Research. 2021 Jan 1;70(1):44-50.

13. Badaeva A, Danilov A, Kosareva A, Lepshina M, Novikov V, Vorobyeva Y, Danilov A. Neuronutritional approach to fibromyalgia management: a narrative review. Pain and Therapy. 2024 Oct;13(5):1047-61.

Chapter 2: The burden of conventional treatments

Fibromyalgia has not lacked for treatment options. Over the last thirty years, both patients and clinicians have had access to an increasing range of treatments including medications, psychological approaches and physical therapies, all of which are supported by varying levels of clinical evidence. The gap between what existing therapies promise and what they actually deliver in practice defines, perhaps more than anything else, the lived experience of fibromyalgia [1,2].

Fibromyalgia impairs every domain of daily life, from the capacity to work and maintain social relationships to the ability to sleep, concentrate, and perform the most ordinary physical tasks [3]. Patients frequently report that their condition is not taken seriously, that treatments are offered without adequate explanation, and that their expectations of improvement are rarely met by what they actually experience [4]. A patient survey examining healthcare experiences in fibromyalgia found that satisfaction with care was low and linked to perceived pain relief, which most patients described as insufficient regardless of the treatment approach [5], reflecting a systemic mismatch between the complexity of the condition and the tools currently available to manage it.

Pharmacological approaches and their limitations

The pharmacological management of fibromyalgia has been shaped by three agents that have received regulatory approval: duloxetine, pregabalin, and milnacipran. Duloxetine and milnacipran are serotonin-norepinephrine reuptake inhibitors, while pregabalin acts on voltage-gated calcium channels to modulate pain signal transmission. All three target aspects of central sensitization and the neurotransmitter imbalances that drive it, and all three have demonstrated statistically significant effects on pain in randomized controlled trials [6,7].

Duloxetine has been the most extensively studied of the three. Systematic reviews and meta-analyses have confirmed that it produces meaningful reductions in pain scores compared to placebo, with additional benefits for mood and overall function [8,9]. Yet the magnitude of these effects is modest. A substantial proportion of patients experience either no meaningful benefit or improvements that fall below what they themselves would consider clinically significant. Tolerability is a persistent concern, with side effects including nausea, somnolence, dry mouth, and sexual dysfunction leading to discontinuation [10]. Pregabalin presents a similar picture, as it reduces pain and improves sleep in some patients, but its sedative properties and association with weight gain limit its long-term acceptability. Milnacipran, while used in some countries, has not achieved the same level of clinical adoption as the other two agents [6,11].

Beyond these three approved agents, a wide range of other medications are used in fibromyalgia, including tricyclic antidepressants, muscle relaxants, opioids, and anticonvulsants. The evidence base for most of these is limited, and the use of opioids in particular has attracted increasing concern. Opioids are generally not recommended in fibromyalgia guidelines because the central sensitization that underlies the condition can be paradoxically worsened by opioid-induced hyperalgesia, a phenomenon in which prolonged opioid use actually increases pain sensitivity rather than reducing it [12]. The picture that emerges is one of partial effects, significant side effect burdens, and a treatment paradigm that addresses symptoms without touching the underlying biology in any meaningful or lasting way [1,7].

The EULAR revised recommendations for fibromyalgia management, which represent the most widely referenced European consensus on the subject, reflect this reality in their conclusions. The guidelines advocate for a stepwise, individualized approach that prioritizes non-pharmacological interventions and reserves drug therapy for specific symptom domains where the evidence is clearest [13]. This represents a significant shift from earlier approaches that placed pharmacotherapy at the center of management.

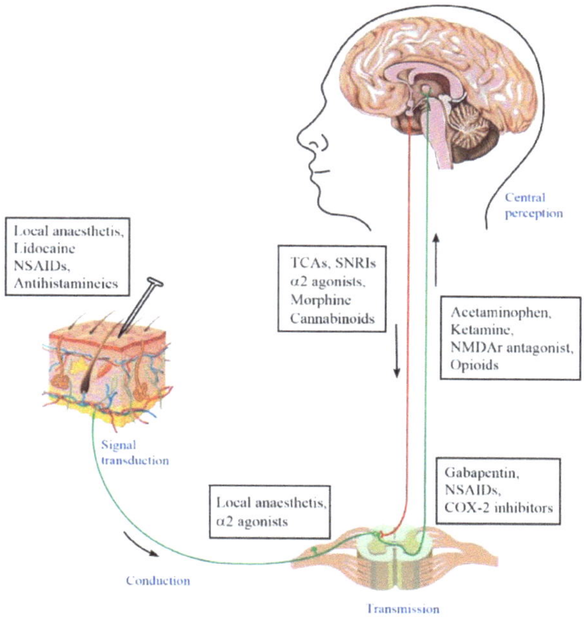

Figure 1*. Pain signal pathways and the sites of action of major pharmacological agents used in fibromyalgia management. Different drug classes act at distinct points along the pain transmission pathway, from signal transduction at the periphery through spinal cord transmission to central perception [14].*

Non-pharmacological interventions

The recognition of fibromyalgia as a multidimensional condition has driven considerable interest in non-pharmacological treatments. Exercise, in particular, has emerged as one of the most consistently effective interventions across multiple systematic reviews and meta-analyses [15,16]. Aerobic exercise, resistance training, and combined programs all show benefits for pain, fatigue, and functional capacity, with effects that compare favorably to pharmacological options in some analyses. The challenge, however, lies in implementation. Patients with fibromyalgia frequently experience post-exertional malaise, meaning that exercise can temporarily worsen symptoms, particularly when programs are introduced too quickly or at too high intensity. Adherence is correspondingly low, and the benefits of exercise depend entirely on sustained participation, which many patients find difficult to maintain over the long term [15,16].

Cognitive behavioral therapy has also accumulated a meaningful evidence base. It is effective in reducing the psychological distress associated with fibromyalgia, improving coping strategies, and reducing the catastrophizing thought patterns that amplify pain perception [17,18]. Acceptance and commitment therapy, a related approach, has shown similar benefits for anxiety and depression in this population. However, cognitive behavioral therapy works at the level of the patient's relationship with their pain rather than at the level of the pain mechanisms themselves. Improvements in psychological outcomes do not always translate into reductions in pain intensity, and patients whose primary complaint is severe physical suffering may find the emphasis on psychological intervention inadequately responsive to what they are actually experiencing [18].

Multimodal treatment programs that combine pharmacological, psychological, and physical approaches have shown the most consistent results in improving quality of life and overall function [19]. Combination approaches have been shown to reduce pain more effectively and improve functional outcomes compared to using a single treatment [19]. This finding is clinically important and highlights a limitation of the current treatment landscape, as achieving good outcomes requires coordinating multiple interventions simultaneously, which in turn demands significant resources, strong patient motivation, and healthcare infrastructure. For many patients, especially those in healthcare systems with limited access to multidisciplinary pain services, the potential benefits of multimodal care are often not accessible in practice [2,20].

The missing piece in fibromyalgia care

Current approaches share a common limitation, as they manage symptoms rather than addressing the underlying biological processes that generate them. Neither pharmacological nor non-pharmacological interventions have demonstrated a capacity to reduce oxidative stress in fibromyalgia patients, restore normal autonomic function, or reverse the neuroplastic changes associated with central sensitization. Patients who respond well to existing treatments often experience partial relief that plateaus after a period of improvement and symptoms often return once treatment is stopped [11,21].

The main challenge in fibromyalgia is not only the need for better drugs or effective exercise programs, but also the need for treatments that address the biological complexity of the condition. The underlying pathophysiology of fibromyalgia is not targeted by current standard of care. Any treatment that go beyond symptom relief needs to directly address these processes and this gap has motivated the exploration of ozone therapy as a potential therapeutic option [22].

Table 1*. Overview of main treatment approaches in fibromyalgia: benefits, limitations, and level of evidence.*

Treatment	Main Benefits	Key Limitations	Evidence
Duloxetine (SNRI)	Pain reduction, mood improvement	Nausea, somnolence, sexual dysfunction, modest effect size	Moderate
Pregabalin	Pain reduction, sleep improvement	Sedation, weight gain, long-term tolerability	Moderate
Milnacipran (SNRI)	Pain reduction	Limited availability, tolerability concerns	Moderate
Exercise therapy	Pain, fatigue, physical function	Poor adherence, post-exertional malaise	Strong
Cognitive behavioral therapy	Mood, coping, anxiety, depression	No direct pain reduction, resource intensive	Moderate
Multimodal treatment	Overall function, quality of life	High resource demand, limited accessibility	Strong

CBT: Cognitive Behavioral Therapy; SNRI: Serotonin-Norepinephrine Reuptake Inhibitor [1,6,13,15,19].

References

1. Giorgi V, Sarzi-Puttini P, Pellegrino G, Sirotti S, Atzeni F, Alciati A, Torta R, Varrassi G, Fornasari D, Coaccioli S, Bongiovanni SF. Pharmacological treatment of fibromyalgia syndrome: a practice-based review. Current Pain and Headache Reports. 2024 Dec;28(12):1349-63.

2. Jurado-Priego LN, Cueto-Ureña C, Ramírez-Expósito MJ, Martínez-Martos JM. Fibromyalgia: a review of the pathophysiological mechanisms and multidisciplinary treatment strategies. Biomedicines. 2024 Jul;12(7):1543.

3. Machado CE, Wendt GW. The impact of fibromyalgia: a cross-sectional examination across different life domains. Journal of Clinical and Translational Research. 2025 Sep 2;11(5):69.

4. Iannuccelli C, Favretti M, Dolcini G, Di Carlo M, Pellegrino G, Bazzichi L, Atzeni F, Lucini D, Varassi G, Leoni ML, Fornasari DM. Fibromyalgia: one year in review 2025. Clinical and Experimental Rheumatology. 2025 Jun 1;43:957-69.

5. Wigers SH, Veierød MB, Mengshoel AM, Forseth KO, Dahli MP, Juel NG, Natvig B. Healthcare experiences of fibromyalgia patients and their associations with satisfaction and pain relief. A patient survey. Scandinavian Journal of Pain. 2024 Apr 16;24(1):20230141.

6. Tzadok R, Ablin JN. Current and emerging pharmacotherapy for fibromyalgia. Pain Research and Management. 2020;2020(1):6541798.

7. Perrot S. Fibromyalgia: do I tackle you with pharmacological treatments? Pain Reports. 2025 Feb 1;10(1):e1222.

8. Lian YN, Wang Y, Zhang Y, Yang CX. Duloxetine for pain in fibromyalgia in adults: a systematic review and a meta-analysis. International Journal of Neuroscience. 2020 Jan 2;130(1):71-82.

9. Migliorini F, Maffulli N, Eschweiler J, Baroncini A, Bell A, Colarossi G. Duloxetine for fibromyalgia syndrome: a systematic review and meta-analysis. Journal of Orthopaedic Surgery and Research. 2023 Jul 17;18(1):504.

10. Rodrigues-Amorim D, Olivares JM, Spuch C, Rivera-Baltanas T. A systematic review of efficacy, safety, and tolerability of duloxetine. Frontiers in Psychiatry. 2020 Oct 23;11:554899.

11. Alorfi NM. Pharmacological treatments of fibromyalgia in adults; overview of phase IV clinical trials. Frontiers in Pharmacology. 2022 Sep 23;13:1017129.

12. Martinez JE, Guimarães I. Fibromyalgia: are there any new approaches? Best Practice and Research Clinical Rheumatology. 2024 Mar 1;38(1):101933.

13. Macfarlane GJ, Kronisch C, Dean LE, Atzeni F, Häuser W, Fluss E, Choy E, Kosek E, Amris K, Branco J, Dincer FI. EULAR revised recommendations for the management of fibromyalgia. Annals of the Rheumatic Diseases. 2017 Feb 1;76(2):318-28.

14. Shinu P, Morsy MA, Nair AB, Mouslem AK, Venugopala KN, Goyal M, Bansal M, Jacob S, Deb PK. Novel therapies for the treatment of neuropathic pain: potential and pitfalls. Journal of Clinical Medicine. 2022 May 26;11(11):3002.

15. Han T, Xi R, Wang J, Yan H, Li L. Adherence to ACSM exercise guidelines and its influence on fibromyalgia treatment outcomes: a meta-analysis of randomized controlled trials. Frontiers in Physiology. 2024 Jul 19;15:1413038.

16. Couto N, Monteiro D, Cid L, Bento T. Effect of different types of exercise in adult subjects with fibromyalgia: a systematic review and meta-analysis of randomised clinical trials. Scientific Reports. 2022 Jun 20;12(1):10391.

17. Heller HL, Borges AR, Franco LO, Aucelio JP, Vargas MI, Lorga RN, Sales MB, Nascimento NV, Netto GF, Passos BC, Paes BP. Role of cognitive behavioral therapy in fibromyalgia: a systematic review. Open Journal of Rheumatology and Autoimmune Diseases. 2021;11(4):169-87.

18. Cojocaru CM, Popa CO, Schenk A, Suciu BA, Szasz S. Cognitive-behavioral therapy and acceptance and commitment therapy for anxiety and depression in patients with fibromyalgia: a systematic review and meta-analysis. Medicine and Pharmacy Reports. 2024 Jan 29;97(1):26.

19. Mascarenhas RO, Souza MB, Oliveira MX, Lacerda AC, Mendonca VA, Henschke N, Oliveira VC. Association of therapies with reduced pain and improved quality of life in patients with fibromyalgia: a systematic review and meta-analysis. JAMA Internal Medicine. 2021 Jan;181(1):104-12.

20. Mettler J, Ming-Azevedo P, Hügle T. Fibromyalgia with concomitant immune-mediated rheumatic diseases: an evaluation of clinical characteristics, diagnostic

criteria and multimodal treatment outcomes. Advances in Rheumatology. 2025 Jun 12;65(1):27.

21. Filipovic T, Filipovic A, Nikolic D, Gimigliano F, Stevanov J, Hrkovic M, Bosanac I. Fibromyalgia: understanding, diagnosis and modern approaches to treatment. Journal of Clinical Medicine. 2025 Feb 2;14(3):955.

22. Clarke H, Peer M, Miles S, Fitzcharles MA. Managing pain in fibromyalgia: current and future options. Drugs. 2025 Sep;85(9):1081-92.

Chapter 3: Ozone therapy — science, history and mechanisms of action

Ozone is not a new discovery, the molecule itself, a triatomic form of oxygen with the chemical formula O3, was first described scientifically in the mid-nineteenth century and its potential applications in biological systems began attracting serious attention not long after. What is relatively new is the depth of understanding that modern molecular biology and biochemistry and how ozone interacts with living tissue and why those interactions can produce effects that are therapeutically relevant rather than simply damaging. The story of ozone in medicine is in many ways the story of learning to distinguish between the molecule as a hazard and the molecule as a tool, and that distinction depends on concentration, context, and the precision with which it is applied [1,2].

The earliest recorded therapeutic uses of ozone date to the late nineteenth and early twentieth centuries, when it was employed as a disinfectant and wound-cleansing agent. Its powerful oxidizing properties made it effective against bacteria, fungi, and viruses, and it found application in the treatment of infected wounds, particularly during the First World War [3]. Over the following decades, interest in its systemic effects grew gradually, as clinicians in Europe, and particularly in Germany, began experimenting with its administration through various routes and observing effects that extended beyond simple antimicrobial action. By the second half of the twentieth century, a body of clinical experience had accumulated that suggested ozone could influence pain, inflammation, and immune function in ways that warranted more rigorous investigation [1,4].

The chemistry of medical ozone

Ozone is an unstable, highly reactive gas that exists in equilibrium with molecular oxygen. Its instability is what gives it biological activity. When ozone comes into contact with biological fluids, it reacts almost immediately with organic compounds and produces a range of secondary molecules that ultimately drive its effects. The most important of these are lipid oxidation products, particularly lipid ozonation products and hydrogen peroxide, which form when ozone reacts with the unsaturated fatty acids present in cell membranes and plasma [5,6]. These secondary messengers are considerably more stable than ozone itself and are capable of diffusing into tissues and cells, where they trigger a range of regulatory responses.

This distinction between ozone as the primary agent and its oxidation products as the biological mediators is fundamental to understanding how ozone therapy works. Ozone does not enter cells directly. What enters cells, and what produces the downstream effects that have been observed clinically, are the lipid peroxidation products and reactive oxygen species generated at the site of ozone contact with biological fluids [7]. The concentration of ozone applied determines the nature and intensity of these effects in a dose-dependent manner. Specifically, at low therapeutic concentrations, the oxidative challenge generated is mild enough to activate adaptive cellular responses without causing damage, while at high concentrations the oxidative load exceeds the capacity of cellular defense systems and produces cytotoxicity. The entire therapeutic rationale of medical ozone rests on operating within the former range, a concept that has been formalized in the literature as oxidative preconditioning [6,8].

Table 1*. Dose-dependent biological effects of medical ozone and their clinical relevance.*

Ozone Concentration	Primary Biological Effect	Cellular Response	Clinical Relevance
Low (10-30 μg/ml)	Mild oxidative stimulus	Nrf2 activation, antioxidant enzyme upregulation	Antioxidant, anti-inflammatory
Medium (30-50 μg/ml)	Moderate oxidative preconditioning	Cytokine modulation, immune regulation	Immunomodulatory, analgesic
High (50-60 μg/ml)	Significant oxidative challenge	Enhanced oxygen metabolism, red cell deformability	Oxygen delivery improvement
Excessive (>60 μg/ml)	Oxidative overload	Cell membrane damage, cytotoxicity	Outside therapeutic range

Adapted from Viebahn-Haensler & León Fernández [6] and Chirumbolo et al. [8]. Therapeutic applications utilize concentrations within the low-to-medium range to activate adaptive responses without cytotoxicity.

The paradox of controlled oxidative stress

The idea that a controlled oxidative challenge could produce antioxidant and anti-inflammatory effects may seem counterintuitive, particularly in a condition like fibromyalgia where oxidative stress is part of the problem rather than the solution.

Resolving this apparent paradox requires an understanding of how cells respond to mild oxidative stimuli.

When cells are exposed to a mild, transient oxidative challenge of the kind produced by low-dose ozone therapy, they activate a set of adaptive responses governed primarily by the transcription factor Nrf2, which functions as the master regulator of the cellular antioxidant defense system [9]. Under normal resting conditions, Nrf2 is kept inactive in the cytoplasm by its inhibitory protein Keap1. When oxidative stress reaches a threshold sufficient to modify specific cysteine residues on Keap1, this inhibition is released, and Nrf2 migrates to the nucleus where it activates the transcription of antioxidant and cytoprotective genes, including superoxide dismutase, catalase, glutathione peroxidase, and heme oxygenase-1 [9,10]. The result of this activation is a significant upregulation of the cell's own antioxidant capacity, an effect that persists well beyond the duration of the initial stimulus.

This mechanism helps explain what is often referred to as the antioxidant paradox, where a treatment that initially introduces oxidative molecules into the body leads, after a short delay, to a measurable reduction in markers of systemic oxidative stress [8,10]. The controlled oxidative challenge acts as a signal rather than a source of damage, training the cellular defense system to operate at a higher level of readiness. In fibromyalgia, where oxidative stress is elevated and antioxidant defenses are demonstrably depleted, this mechanism offers a rationale for therapeutic intervention that is mechanistically coherent rather than empirically speculative. The ozone-induced upregulation of antioxidant enzymes directly addresses one of the core biological abnormalities identified in the condition [6,9].

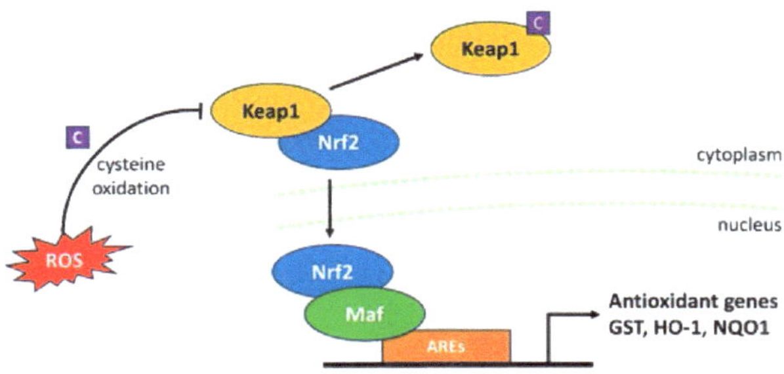

***Figure 1**. Schematic representation of the Nrf2-Keap1-ARE signaling pathway. ROS-induced cysteine oxidation on Keap1 releases Nrf2, which translocates to the nucleus and activates antioxidant defense genes including GST, HO-1, and NQO1 [9,11].*

Anti-inflammatory and immune-modulating effects

Beyond its effects on oxidative balance, ozone therapy has been shown to exert significant influences on inflammatory pathways and immune function. The lipid oxidation products generated by ozone-biological fluid interactions act as signaling molecules that modulate the production and activity of cytokines, the small proteins that coordinate the inflammatory response. In particular, repeated low-dose ozone exposure has been associated with reductions in pro-inflammatory cytokines such as interleukin-1 beta, interleukin-6, and tumor necrosis factor-alpha, alongside increases in anti-inflammatory mediators [5,7]. These changes are not immediate but develop progressively with repeated treatments, consistent with the idea that ozone acts through adaptive signaling pathways.

Ozone therapy has been also shown to modulate the activity of immune cells, including macrophages and lymphocytes, in ways that shift the overall immune environment away from a pro-inflammatory state [12,13]. This immunomodulatory capacity is particularly significant because fibromyalgia involves not only peripheral sensitization and central nervous system dysregulation but also low-grade systemic inflammation that conventional treatments do not address directly [14].

Effects on oxygen metabolism and mitochondrial function

One of the most clinically relevant properties of medical ozone is its ability to improve oxygen delivery and utilization at the cellular level. Ozone therapy increases the deformability of red blood cells, allowing them to pass more easily through the small capillaries that supply peripheral tissues, and it enhances the release of oxygen from hemoglobin by stimulating the production of 2,3-diphosphoglycerate [1,5]. The result is improved tissue oxygenation, which has direct implications for the mitochondrial dysfunction that contributes to fatigue and musculoskeletal symptoms in fibromyalgia. When mitochondria receive adequate oxygen supply, their capacity to generate ATP through oxidative phosphorylation improves, and the production of excess reactive oxygen species as a byproduct of impaired energy metabolism is reduced [6,15].

This improvement in cellular energy metabolism represents another point at which ozone therapy engages directly with the underlying biology of fibromyalgia rather than simply managing its symptoms. The fatigue that fibromyalgia patients experience is not a psychological consequence of chronic pain, but it has a metabolic basis in the form of mitochondrial dysfunction and interventions that restore more normal mitochondrial function address this dimension of the condition at its source [15].

Safety profile and the importance of concentration

Any discussion of ozone therapy needs to address safety, especially since ozone is known to be harmful when inhaled as an air pollutant. The key point is that medical use is very different from environmental exposure, as ozone in a clinical setting is applied in controlled concentrations and is not given by inhalation [2,4]. Medical ozone is generated on demand using certified equipment that produces ozone-oxygen mixtures at defined concentrations, expressed in micrograms of ozone per milliliter of gas, and the therapeutic range for systemic applications lies well below the concentrations associated with tissue damage [1,16].

When used within established therapeutic parameters, ozone therapy has demonstrated a favorable safety profile, as adverse effects are uncommon, mild and serious complications are rare in properly conducted treatments [14,16]. The nature of ozone's biological effects, whereby low doses produce adaptive and protective responses while high doses produce toxicity, is well supported by experimental evidence and provides a scientific basis for the careful dose management that characterizes responsible clinical practice [12]. The growing body of research on ozone therapy in musculoskeletal pain conditions, including its application specifically in chronic pain syndromes, reflects an increasing confidence in its safety [14,16].

References

1. Hidalgo-Tallón FJ, Torres-Morera LM, Baeza-Noci J, Carrillo-Izquierdo MD, Pinto-Bonilla R. Updated review on ozone therapy in pain medicine. Frontiers in Physiology. 2022 Feb 23;13:840623.

2. Alvim-Ferraz MC, Sousa SI, Martins FG, Ferraz MP. Tropospheric and stratospheric ozone: scientific history and shifts in early perspectives regarding the impact on human health. Atmosphere. 2024 Dec 17;15(12):1504.

3. Zhang K, Liu J, Lv H, Zeng X, Ling Z, Ding L, Jin C. Advances in ozone technology for environmental, energy, food and medical applications. Processes. 2025 Apr 9;13(4):1126.

4. Serra ME, Baeza-Noci J, Mendes Abdala CV, Luvisotto MM, Bertol CD, Anzolin AP. The role of ozone treatment as integrative medicine. An evidence and gap map. Frontiers in Public Health. 2023 Jan 16;10:1112296.

5. Smith NL, Wilson AL, Gandhi J, Vatsia S, Khan SA. Ozone therapy: an overview of pharmacodynamics, current research, and clinical utility. Medical Gas Research. 2017 Jul 1;7(3):212-9.

6. Viebahn-Haensler R, León Fernández OS. Ozone as redox bioregulator in preventive medicine: the molecular and pharmacological basis of the low-dose ozone concept — a review. International Journal of Molecular Sciences. 2023 Oct 30;24(21):15747.

7. Cernei N, Sandru S, Cobiletchi S, Grabovschi I, Civirjic I, Baltaga R. Current affairs in the use of medical ozone. Biological effects. Mechanisms of action. Revista de Stiinte ale Sanatatii din Moldova. 2023 Sep 28(3):65-72.

8. Chirumbolo S, Tirelli U, Franzini M, Pandolfi S, Ricevuti G, Vaiano F, Valdenassi L. Ozone in the adjunct medical treatment. The round personality of a molecule with hormetic properties. Human and Experimental Toxicology. 2023 Nov 22;42:09603271231218926.

9. Galie M, Covi V, Tabaracci G, Malatesta M. The role of Nrf2 in the antioxidant cellular response to medical ozone exposure. International Journal of Molecular Sciences. 2019 Aug 17;20(16):4009.

11. Hong Y, Boiti A, Vallone D, Foulkes NS. Reactive oxygen species signaling and oxidative stress: transcriptional regulation and evolution. Antioxidants. 2024 Mar 1;13(3):312.

10. Sanjaya IN, Andonotopo W, Bachnas MA, Dewantiningrum J, Pramono MB, Darmawan E, Aldiansyah D, Stanojevic M, Kurjak A. Therapeutic ozone in preeclamptic pregnancy: mechanistic insights, clinical gaps, and the oxidative paradox. Medicine Research and Clinical Practice. 2025 Apr 1;2(2):27-37.

12. Malatesta M, Cisterna B, Costanzo M. Cellular and molecular mechanisms of ozone therapy: present knowledge and prospective applications. International Journal of Molecular Sciences. 2022 Oct 20;23(20):12586.

13. El Meligy OA, Elemam NM, Talaat IM. Ozone therapy in medicine and dentistry: a review of the literature. Dentistry Journal. 2023 Aug 7;11(8):187.

14. de Araujo LT, da Silva PC, Masini M. Medical ozone as a therapeutic option in musculoskeletal pain control: a critical review of clinical trials considering safety and quality indicators for procedures and devices. The Yale Journal of Biology and Medicine. 2024 Sep 30;97(3):383.

15. Wang S, Li M, Liu Y, Chen C, Yang F. Mechanisms and clinical applications of ozone and ozonated oil as antimicrobial systems. Journal of Materials Chemistry B. 2026.

16. Sumida JM, Hayashi AM. Ozone therapy in veterinary medicine: clinical indications and techniques. Acta Veterinaria Brasilica. 2022 Dec 9;16(4):294-304.

Chapter 4: Major Autohemotherapy

Among the different ways ozone has been used in medicine, major autohemotherapy has a central role, as it has the longest clinical use, the strongest body of evidence, and a clearly defined way of being performed. Most of what is known about the biological effects of ozone comes from research on this method. Understanding how major autohemotherapy works, how it is carried out, and how it affects the blood and the body is important when considering its role in fibromyalgia [1,2].

The concept of autohemotherapy predates the clinical use of ozone by several decades. The practice of withdrawing a patient's own blood, treating it in some way, and reinfusing it has roots in early twentieth century medicine, where it was used in various forms to stimulate immune responses and promote healing. The incorporation of ozone into this framework emerged as part of the broader development of ozone medicine in Europe, and by the mid-twentieth century the combination of blood withdrawal, ozone treatment, and reinfusion had been formalized into what is now described as major autohemotherapy to distinguish it from minor autohemotherapy, a simpler procedure involving much smaller volumes [2,3]. Major autohemotherapy operates on a scale that produces measurable systemic effects, making it a genuinely therapeutic [1].

The choice of blood as the vehicle for ozone delivery reflects a fundamental insight about the molecule's biological behavior. Ozone does not exert its effects directly but through the secondary products generated when it reacts with biological substrates. Blood, with its rich content of lipids, proteins, and cellular components, provides precisely the reactive environment needed to convert an ozone-oxygen gas mixture into a set of biologically active molecules. When ozone is introduced into a volume of blood outside the body, the reaction is rapid, and reproducible, producing a defined profile of lipid oxidation products and reactive oxygen species that, upon reinfusion, distribute throughout the body and trigger the cellular responses that constitute the therapeutic effect [4,5].

The Procedure: From Blood Draw to Reinfusion

The procedure of major autohemotherapy follows a clearly defined sequence that, when carried out under appropriate conditions, is simple and reproducible. A volume of venous blood, typically between 100 and 200 milliliters, is withdrawn from the patient into a sterile, closed glass or plastic container that has been prepared with an anticoagulant to prevent clotting during the treatment phase. The container is then connected to an ozone generator, which introduces a precise volume of an ozone-oxygen gas mixture into the blood at a defined concentration. The ozone concentration used for systemic applications generally falls within the range of 20 to 40 micrograms per milliliter of gas, though the specific parameters vary depending on the clinical indication, the patient's condition, and the protocol being followed [1,6]. The blood and ozone-oxygen mixture are gently combined, usually by swirling or inverting the container to ensure thorough contact between the gas and the blood without mechanical damage to the cellular components. Once the reaction is complete, the treated blood is reinfused intravenously into the patient through the same access point used for the initial withdrawal [7,8].

The entire procedure typically takes between thirty and sixty minutes, is performed in an outpatient setting, and requires no anesthesia or recovery period. Patients remain seated or recumbent throughout and are generally able to resume normal activities immediately afterward. The number of sessions prescribed varies with the clinical context, but treatment courses of ten to twenty sessions administered two to three times per week are commonly described in the literature and reflect the understanding that the biological effects of ozone therapy are cumulative and develop progressively over the course of a treatment cycle [6,9]. The interval between sessions is as important as the sessions themselves, as it allows the adaptive cellular responses triggered by each treatment to develop and consolidate before the next oxidative stimulus is applied [5,10].

The equipment used in major autohemotherapy is specialized and subject to quality standards that are fundamental to procedural safety. Medical ozone generators produce ozone by passing pure medical-grade oxygen through an electrical discharge, and the resulting ozone-oxygen mixture is delivered at concentrations that are precisely measured and calibrated. The use of pure oxygen as the carrier gas is essential, as air contains nitrogen that can form toxic nitrogen oxides when exposed to an electrical discharge, which is why it is not used in ozone therapy [11]. Equally important is the use of ozone-resistant materials for all tubing and containers that are in contact with the gas, as ozone rapidly degrades standard plastics and rubber. These technical requirements highlight the importance of proper training and certified equipment in clinical practice [9,12].

The Blood's Response to Ozone Treatment

The contact between ozone and blood during major autohemotherapy initiates a lot of changes in the blood's cellular and molecular components that define the treatment's biological profile. Additionally, erythrocytes in fibromyalgia patients, as in many chronic pain conditions, show reduced deformability, meaning they are less able to change shape as needed to pass through the narrow capillaries that supply peripheral tissues. This rigidity impairs microcirculation and contributes to the tissue hypoxia that may underlie some of the musculoskeletal symptoms patients experience. Ozone treatment has been shown to reverse this pattern, significantly improving erythrocyte deformability and reducing the aggregation tendency that compounds microcirculatory impairment [13,14,15]. These changes lead to improved tissue perfusion and better oxygen delivery to muscles and other peripheral tissues.

The effects of ozone on hemoglobin, the protein responsible for oxygen transport within red blood cells, add a further dimension to this improvement in oxygen delivery. At the molecular level, controlled ozonation of blood has been shown to modify the structural and functional properties of hemoglobin enhancing its capacity to release oxygen to peripheral tissues. The 2,3-diphosphoglycerate pathway, which regulates the affinity of hemoglobin for oxygen and determines how readily oxygen is released to cells, is stimulated by the mild oxidative conditions produced during major autohemotherapy [16,17]. The practical consequence is a shift in the oxygen-hemoglobin dissociation curve, meaning that hemoglobin releases oxygen more readily at the tissue level, an effect that is needed in conditions characterized by peripheral tissue hypoxia and impaired energy metabolism. Research has also shown that the antioxidant status of the blood at the time of ozonation influences how hemoglobin responds, which highlights the importance of adequate nutritional antioxidant support in patients undergoing ozone therapy [16].

In addition, ozone treatment during major autohemotherapy exerts significant effects on the immune cells circulating in the blood. Platelets, which play a role not only in coagulation but also in the modulation of inflammatory responses, show altered activation patterns following ozone treatment, with changes that contribute to the reduction in low-grade systemic inflammation [17,18]. White blood cells, including lymphocytes, monocytes, and neutrophils, respond to the mild oxidative stimulus of ozone contact by activating signaling pathways that influence their behavior after reinfusion. It has been shown that ozone exposure modulates the viability and functional activity of neutrophils and monocytes in ways consistent with a shift toward a less pro-inflammatory phenotype, an effect that has been observed across different experimental models and appears to be concentration-dependent [19,20].

The relationship between ozone treatment and the immune system extends beyond these immediate cellular changes. Ozone-treated blood releases the lipid oxidation products generated during the extracorporeal treatment phase into the systemic circulation, where they act as signaling molecules capable of modulating immune function throughout the body. This mechanism, often described as a form of autovaccination, uses the body's own immune regulatory pathways to shift the inflammatory balance, with repeated exposure to mild oxidative stimuli through sessions of major autohemotherapy leading to a gradual adjustment of immune responses that develops over the course of treatment and persist beyond its completion [18,21].

Systemic Effects: Circulation, Metabolism and the Autonomic Nervous System

The systemic effects of major autohemotherapy include changes in circulatory, metabolic, and neurological function that are relevant to the fibromyalgia syndrome. One of the most commonly reported systemic effects is improved microcirculation, driven by better erythrocyte deformability, enhanced oxygen release from hemoglobin, and vasodilation linked to ozone-related changes in nitric oxide metabolism. The result is a measurable improvement in tissue oxygenation that affects not only skeletal muscle but also organs and tissues throughout the body [22,3]. In fibromyalgia, where impaired peripheral circulation and tissue hypoxia contribute to fatigue and myalgia, this improvement in oxygen delivery represents a meaningful therapeutic effect.

The metabolic consequences of major autohemotherapy complement its circulatory effects in important ways. Improved tissue oxygenation supports more efficient mitochondrial function, reducing the accumulation of lactate and other metabolic byproducts that contribute to muscle pain and fatigue. At the same time, the upregulation of antioxidant defenses triggered by the ozone-induced Nrf2 pathway reduces the mitochondrial oxidative damage that impairs energy production at the cellular level. The overall effect is a shift toward a more efficient and less harmful metabolic environment in peripheral tissues, addressing one of the biological factors behind fibromyalgia fatigue that conventional pharmacological treatments do not affect [10,17].

One of the most relevant systemic effects of major autohemotherapy in fibromyalgia is its influence on the autonomic nervous system. Autonomic dysregulation, characterized by sympathetic overactivation and reduced parasympathetic tone, is a well-recognized feature of fibromyalgia that contributes to sleep disturbances, cardiovascular variability, and the amplification of pain responses. Repeated ozone therapy has been associated with a measurable shift in autonomic balance toward greater parasympathetic tone, an effect that may normalize some of the autonomic abnormalities [22,1]. This influence on autonomic function also has implications for the pain-sleep cycle, since improved autonomic regulation supports more restorative sleep, which in turn reduces the central sensitization.

Safety, Guidelines and Clinical Protocols

The clinical application of major autohemotherapy is guided by guidelines and protocols developed over decades of practice and refined through the work of international bodies dedicated to ozone medicine. The International Scientific Committee of Ozone Therapy (ISCO3) has published guidelines that define the technical requirements for ozone generation, the therapeutic concentration ranges for different indications, the procedural standards for blood handling, and the training requirements for practitioners [9]. These guidelines reflect a clear understanding that safety and effectiveness of ozone therapy depend on how precisely it is applied, and that deviations from established protocols, whether through excessive concentrations, inappropriate routes of administration, or inadequate equipment, introduce risks that can be avoided [11,12].

The contraindications to major autohemotherapy are few but should be observed carefully. Severe anemia and conditions associated with abnormal coagulation represent relative contraindications, as does hyperthyroidism, given ozone's stimulatory effects on metabolic rate. Glucose-6-phosphate dehydrogenase deficiency is a specific contraindication because this enzyme deficiency impairs the cell's ability to regenerate the reduced glutathione needed to manage the oxidative challenge of ozone treatment. Pregnancy, severe thrombocytopenia, and active hemorrhage are also contraindications [12,23]. The administration of ozone intravenously as a pure gas, without first mixing it with blood, is absolutely prohibited under all clinical protocols, as gaseous embolism under these conditions can be fatal. Rectal, vaginal, topical, and other localized routes of administration each have their own specific considerations, but when major autohemotherapy is performed according to established protocols, it has shown a consistent record of safety over time [11,9].

How ozone therapy is viewed by healthcare professionals reflects a broader difficulty in bringing less conventional but evidence based approaches into routine practice. Knowledge of how it works and how it is used varies and many clinicians have had little formal exposure to it during their training [24]. This gap is significant because the appropriate and safe application of major autohemotherapy depends on knowledge of its technical requirements and its clinical indications, and misinformation in either direction ultimately disadvantages the patients who might benefit from it. The range of ozone therapy's applications, extending from musculoskeletal conditions to dermatological disorders and even veterinary medicine, reflects both its versatility and the need for clear guidance [25,26].

Evidence in Fibromyalgia: From Pilot Studies to Clinical Data

The application of major autohemotherapy specifically in fibromyalgia has been the subject of a growing number of clinical investigations, ranging from early pilot studies to more recent prospective and retrospective analyses. One of the earlier dedicated studies of major ozone autohemotherapy in fibromyalgia reported significant improvements in pain scores and physical functionality following a structured treatment course. Patients who received major autohemotherapy showed reductions in pain index and improvements in quality of life that were statistically significant and clearly noticeable in clinical practice [27]. A prospective cross-sectional study confirmed these findings, demonstrating improvements in physical functionality and overall quality of life in fibromyalgia patients treated with major ozone autohemotherapy, with changes in pain intensity that compared to outcomes reported with pharmacological interventions in similar populations [28]. More recently, a retrospective clinical study examining the effects of major ozone autohemotherapy in a larger group of fibromyalgia patients reported significant reductions in pain, fatigue, and sleep disturbances, with a favorable tolerability profile and no serious adverse events [29].

Taken together, these clinical observations align well with the underlying mechanistic framework. The improvements in pain, fatigue, and sleep quality that fibromyalgia patients experience following major autohemotherapy are consistent with what would be expected from a treatment that simultaneously reduces oxidative stress, improves peripheral tissue oxygenation, modulates pro-inflammatory cytokine profiles, and supports autonomic rebalancing. None of these effects is peripheral to the condition being treated, but aach one addresses a dimension of fibromyalgia pathophysiology. The available clinical data, although still limited, fit within a clear mechanistic understanding that reflects the underlying biology of the condition, while further research, especially larger and well designed studies, is needed to better define how consistent these effects are across different patients [27,28,29].

References

1. Viebahn-Hänsler R, León Fernández OS, Fahmy Z. Ozone in medicine: clinical evaluation and evidence classification of the systemic ozone applications, major autohemotherapy and rectal insufflation, according to the requirements for evidence-based medicine. Ozone: Science and Engineering. 2016;38(5):322-45.

2. Maslennikov OV, Kontorshchikova CN, Gribkova IA. Ozone therapy in practice. Health Manual, Ministry Health Service of The Russian Federation, The State Medical Academy of Nizhny Novgorod, Russia. 2008.

3. Di Paolo N, Bocci V, Gaggiotti E. Ozone therapy. The International Journal of Artificial Organs. 2004;27(3):168-75.

4. Travagli V, Zanardi I, Bocci V. A realistic evaluation of the action of ozone on whole human blood. International Journal of Biological Macromolecules. 2006;39(4-5):317-20.

5. Tricarico G, Travagli V. The relationship between ozone and human blood in the course of a well-controlled, mild, and transitory oxidative eustress. Antioxidants. 2021;10(12):1946.

6. Viebahn-Hänsler R, León Fernández OS, Fahmy Z. Ozone in medicine: the low-dose ozone concept — guidelines and treatment strategies. Ozone: Science and Engineering. 2012;34(6):408-24.

7. Smith NL, Wilson AL, Gandhi J, Vatsia S, Khan SA. Ozone therapy: an overview of pharmacodynamics, current research, and clinical utility. Medical Gas Research. 2017;7(3):212-9.

8. Re L, Rowen R, Travagli V. Ozone therapy and its use in medicine: further comments. Cardiology. 2017;136(4):269.

9. Konrad H. International Scientific Committee of Ozone Therapy ISCO3. 2014.

10. Altman N. The new oxygen prescription: the miracle of oxidative therapies. Simon and Schuster. 2017.

13. Akbudak IH, Kucukatay V, Kilic-Erkek O, Ozdemir Y, Bor-Kucukatay M. Investigation of the effects of major ozone autohemotherapy application on erythrocyte deformability and aggregation. Clinical Hemorheology and Microcirculation. 2019;71(3):365-72.

14. Seda Artis A, Aydogan S, Gokhan Sahin M. The effects of colorectally insufflated oxygen-ozone on red blood cell rheology in rabbits. Clinical Hemorheology and Microcirculation. 2010;45(2-4):329-36.

15. Deryugina AV, Boyarinov GA, Simutis IS, Nikolskiy VO, Kuznetsov AB, Efimova TS. Correction of metabolic indicators of erythrocytes and myocardium structure with ozonized red blood-cell mass. Cell and Tissue Biology. 2018;12(3):207-12.

16. Mehraban F, Seyedarabi A, Seraj Z, Ahmadian S, Poursasan N, Rayati S, Moosavi-Movahedi AA. Molecular insights into the effect of ozone on human hemoglobin in autohemotherapy: highlighting the importance of the presence of blood antioxidants during ozonation. International Journal of Biological Macromolecules. 2018;119:1276-85.

17. Di Paolo N, Gaggiotti E, Galli F. Extracorporeal blood oxygenation and ozonation: clinical and biological implications of ozone therapy. Redox Report. 2005;10(3):121-30.

18. Chirumbolo S, Valdenassi L, Tirelli U, Ricevuti G, Pandolfi S, Vaiano F, Franzini M. The oxygen-ozone adjunct medical treatment according to the protocols from the Italian Scientific Society of Oxygen-Ozone Therapy: how ozone applications in the blood can influence clinical therapy success via the modulation of cell biology and immunity. Biology. 2023;12(12):1512.

19. Frush BW, Li Z, Stiles JV, Cotter SF, Shofer SL, Foster WM, Tighe RM. Ozone primes alveolar macrophage-derived innate immunity in healthy human subjects. Journal of Allergy and Clinical Immunology. 2016;138(4):1213-15.

20. Nguyen Ngoc D, Valverde Piedra JL, Milczak A, Szponder T, Drzewiecka B, Pyzerska A, Wessely-Szponder J. Mild ozone-induced oxidative stress modulates the activity and viability of porcine neutrophils and monocytes. Animals. 2026;16(2):193.

21. Ogut E. Mechanisms and therapeutic potential of ozone therapy in enhancing vasculogenesis and angiogenesis through growth factor activation and oxidative signaling pathways. Discover Medicine. 2025;2(1):240.

22. Hidalgo-Tallón FJ, Torres-Morera LM, Baeza-Noci J, Carrillo-Izquierdo MD, Pinto-Bonilla R. Updated review on ozone therapy in pain medicine. Frontiers in Physiology. 2022;13:840623.

11. Sánchez GM, Tapia AS, Mariño RQ, Sabbah F. Non-recommended routes of application in ozone therapy, a critical review. Ozone Therapy Global Journal. 2018;8(1):19-35.

12. Bocci V. Side effects and contraindications of ozonetherapy. In: Oxygen-Ozone Therapy: A Critical Evaluation. Dordrecht: Springer Netherlands; 2002. p. 227-31.

23. de los Ángeles Erario M, Grangeat AM. Medical ozone treatments: the good, the bad, and the ugly. Journal of Orthopedics. 2025;17(2).

24. Yazicioglu B, Oruc MA, Emin Goktepe M, Ozturk O. Knowledge and attitude of healthcare professionals towards ozone therapy. Alternative Therapies in Health and Medicine. 2023;29(7):238-41.

25. Modena DAO, de Castro Ferreira R, Froes PM, Rocha KC. Ozone therapy for dermatological conditions: a systematic review. The Journal of Clinical and Aesthetic Dermatology. 2022;15(5):65.

26. Sumida JM, Hayashi AM. Ozone therapy in veterinary medicine: clinical indications and techniques. Acta Veterinaria Brasilica. 2022;16(4):294-304.

27. Ahi ED, Afsar SI. The effectiveness of major ozone autohemotherapy in the treatment of fibromyalgia syndrome. Journal of Surgery and Medicine. 2022;6(8):746-50.

28. Türkyılmaz GG, Rumeli S, Bakır M. Effects of major ozone autohemotherapy on physical functionality and quality of life in fibromyalgia syndrome: a prospective cross-sectional study. Alternative Therapies in Health and Medicine. 2021;27(5):8-12.

29. Çiftci İnceoğlu S, Ayyıldız A, Erden MF, Asik M, İnceoğlu A, Kuran B. Effects of major ozone autohemotherapy on fibromyalgia: a retrospective clinical study. Egyptian Rheumatology and Rehabilitation. 2026;53(1):16.

Chapter 5: The Role of Autohemotherapy with Ozone as an Effective Treatment for Fibromyalgia – Clinical Study

This chapter presents the clinical study that forms the foundation of this book, which is a prospective observational study conducted to evaluate the effectiveness of major autohemotherapy with ozone in patients diagnosed with fibromyalgia, presented at the European Society of Regional Anaesthesia and Pain Therapy (ESRA) Annual Congress in 2024 [1]. The study was driven by the fact that patients with fibromyalgia still have limited effective treatment options, and by the idea that ozone therapy can act on several key biological processes of the condition at the same time, something that conventional treatments have not been able to do consistently.

Study Design and Methods

Twenty patients with a confirmed diagnosis of fibromyalgia were enrolled in the study, all of whom provided informed consent prior to participation. The study was conducted with ethics committee approval. The patient group had a mean age of 50 years and comprised equal numbers of men and women. The mean duration of disease from the time of diagnosis was two years, reflecting a population in the established but not end-stage phase of the condition, where the biological processes driving symptoms are active and measurable but the disease has not yet undergone the chronification that might be expected to reduce treatment responsiveness.

Each patient received ten sessions of major ozone autohemotherapy, administered at a frequency of two sessions per week, for five weeks. The ozone-oxygen mixture was applied at concentrations ranging from 30 to 60 micrograms per milliliter, within the established therapeutic range for systemic ozone applications. The procedure followed the standard major autohemotherapy protocol, where venous blood was withdrawn into a sterile closed container, mixed with the ozone-oxygen gas mixture under controlled conditions, and then reinfused intravenously into the patient. No adverse events of any kind were recorded during the treatment period [1].

The primary outcome measures were pain intensity, assessed using the Visual Analog Scale (VAS), and the frequency of fibromyalgia flares. The VAS is a validated and widely used instrument in fibromyalgia research that asks patients to rate their pain on a scale from 0 to 10, where 0 represents no pain and 10 represents the worst imaginable pain (Figure 1). Assessments were conducted immediately before the first session and after the completion of the tenth session. The number of tender points and patients' self-reported quality of sleep and capacity to perform everyday activities were also recorded throughout the treatment course [1].

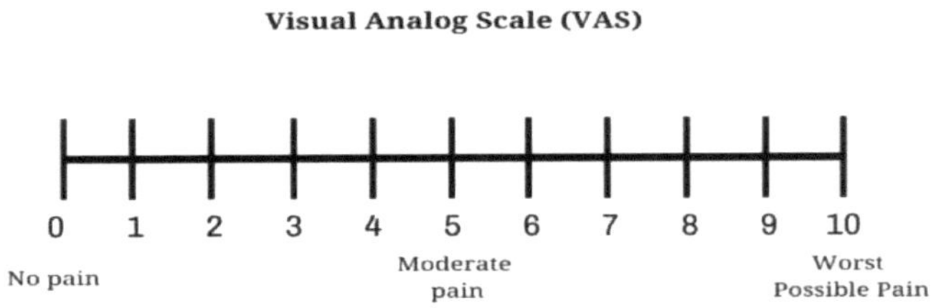

Figure 1. *The Visual Analog Scale (VAS) used to assess pain intensity. Patients rate their pain from 0 (no pain) to 10 (worst possible pain).*

Results

The results were consistent across the entire patient group. Every one of the twenty patients who completed the treatment course reported an improvement in their condition following the ten sessions of major autohemotherapy. This consistent response is clinically important, as patients with fibromyalgia usually respond differently to treatment, and conventional drugs tend to help only some of them.

Pain intensity, as measured by the VAS, decreased in all twenty patients. The mean VAS score before treatment was 8.7, reflecting the severe pain burden characteristic of this patient population. Following the completion of ten ozone autohemotherapy sessions, the mean VAS score fell to 5.9, representing a mean reduction of 2.8 points, equivalent to approximately 32 percent from baseline. Of the twenty patients, eighteen showed a reduction of two or more VAS points, and ten showed a reduction of three or more points. Before treatment, all twenty patients were in the severe pain category (VAS 7 or above), while after treatment, thirteen patients had shifted to the moderate pain range (VAS 4 to 6), and the proportion of patients with severe pain fell from 100 percent to 35 percent. The descriptive statistics and pain category distribution are summarized in Table 1 and individual patient data are presented in Table 2.

Table 1. Summary statistics of VAS scores before and after ten sessions of ozone autohemotherapy (n=20) [1].

	VAS Before Treatment	VAS After Treatment	Reduction
Mean	8.7	5.9	2.8
Median	9.0	6.0	3.0
Standard Deviation	0.54	1.22	1.23
Minimum	8.0	4.0	0.5
Maximum	10.0	9.0	5.0
Patients with severe pain (VAS ≥7)	20/20 (100%)	7/20 (35%)	
Patients with moderate pain (VAS 4-6)	0/20 (0%)	13/20 (65%)	

VAS: Visual Analog Scale (0 = no pain, 10 = worst imaginable pain). Severe pain defined as VAS ≥7; moderate pain as VAS 4-6.

Beyond pain, all twenty patients described a marked decrease in the frequency of fibromyalgia flares, the episodic worsening of symptoms that significantly disrupts daily functioning and represents one of the most disabling aspects of the condition. The frequency of flares decreased by approximately 50 percent during the course of treatment, a reduction that patients themselves described as having a meaningful impact on their ability to plan and sustain everyday activities. A reduction in the number of tender points was also observed across the patient group. Perhaps most meaningful in terms of quality of life were the improvements in sleep and in the ability to carry out everyday activities reported by all patients. Sleep, which is both severely impaired in fibromyalgia and a key driver of central sensitization, showed notable improvement following the treatment course, and patients described a greater ability to engage in routine daily activities that had previously been limited by pain and fatigue [1].

A further finding of practical importance was the observation that the treatment reduced patients' reliance on analgesic medications. Fibromyalgia patients frequently depend on daily pain medication, which carries its own burden in terms of side effects and long-term tolerability. The reduction in medication use reported by patients following ozone autohemotherapy suggests that the therapy's benefits extended beyond direct symptom relief to include a broader improvement in the patient's overall therapeutic situation [1].

***Table 2**. Individual Visual Analog Scale (VAS) scores before and after ten sessions of ozone autohemotherapy [1].*

Patient	VAS Before	VAS After	Patient	VAS Before	VAS After
1	9-10	5-6	11	9	7
2	8	6	12	8	5
3	8	5	13	8	7
4	9-10	7	14	9	7
5	8-9	4	15	9	6
6	8	6	16	8	5
7	9	7	17	9	7
8	9	5	18	9	6
9	9	4	19	9	4
10	8	6	20	9	8-9
Mean	**8.7**	**5.9**			

VAS: Visual Analog Scale (0 = no pain, 10 = worst imaginable pain). Ranges indicate patient-reported variability at assessment.

Discussion

The findings of this study are consistent with the growing body of clinical evidence supporting ozone therapy in fibromyalgia. A randomized double-blind placebo-controlled study similarly found statistically significant reductions in pain intensity and Fibromyalgia Impact Questionnaire scores following major autohemotherapy, confirming that the improvements observed are not attributable to placebo response [2]. In addition, a large case series examining outcomes in two hundred fibromyalgia patients treated with oxygen-ozone autohemotherapy reported clinically meaningful pain reductions in the majority of patients, a finding broadly consistent with the universal improvement observed in the present study [3]. Earlier randomized controlled evidence also demonstrated superior outcomes with ozone therapy compared to control conditions in fibromyalgia patients [4].

What distinguishes the present study within this body of evidence is the breadth of its outcome assessment. The observation that all twenty patients reported simultaneous improvements in pain, sleep quality, daily activity capacity, tender points, and flare frequency is consistent with the multidimensional mode of action that ozone therapy exerts, acting on oxidative stress, inflammatory pathways, oxygen metabolism, and autonomic regulation simultaneously. This pattern of improvement across multiple symptoms stands in contrast to the more limited and often partial benefits seen with conventional pharmacological treatments.

The study has limitations that should be acknowledged. The absence of a control group means that the contribution of placebo effects to the observed improvements cannot be formally excluded, though the consistency of the response across all twenty patients and its alignment with controlled trial evidence from other groups provides meaningful reassurance. The sample size of twenty patients, while appropriate for an initial clinical evaluation, limits the statistical precision of the findings. Follow-up data after the end of treatment were not available, so the duration of the observed improvements remains uncertain. This highlights the need for further research, particularly larger controlled studies with longer follow-up periods.

References

1. Dimou T. LP004 The role of autohemotherapy with ozone as an effective treatment for fibromyalgia. European Society of Regional Anaesthesia and Pain Therapy (ESRA) Annual Congress; 2024. DOI: 10.1136/rapm-2024-ESRA.589.

2. Sucuoğlu H, Soydaş N. Efficacy of ozone therapy as an add-on treatment in fibromyalgia: a randomized double-blind placebo-controlled study. Journal of Back and Musculoskeletal Rehabilitation. 2023;36(2):357-66.

3. Tirelli U, Franzini M, Valdenassi L, Pandolfi S, Taibi R, Chirumbolo S. Fibromyalgia treated with oxygen-ozone auto-haemotherapy (O2-O3-AHT): a case study on 200 patients with a modified 10-PI-NRS evaluation. European Review for Medical and Pharmacological Sciences. 2022;26(21).

4. Fahmy Z. Controlled study of the efficacy ozone therapy in fibromyalgia, a randomised controlled trial. Journal of Ozone Therapy. 2019;3(4):20.

Chapter 6: Discussion, Clinical Evidence and Future Directions

The results of this study carry a significance that extends beyond the patients who participated in it. In fibromyalgia, a condition that has resisted many therapeutic attempts over the decades, finding that every patient in a treatment group improves across several symptom areas at the same time is genuinely uncommon. Tthe consistency of the response observed in this study is worth examining carefully, in order to understand what it suggests when placed alongside the growing body of evidence that has been building in this field.

A mean reduction of 2.8 points on the Visual Analog Scale, from 8.7 to 5.9, represents a clinically meaningful improvement. In fibromyalgia research, a reduction of two or more points on the VAS is regarded as clinically important, reflecting a level of improvement that patients can perceive in their daily experience of pain. In this study, eighteen of the twenty patients reached that threshold. There was also a clear shift in pain severity, while before treatment, all patients were in the severe pain range. After ten sessions of major autohemotherapy, thirteen had moved to the moderate range, and the proportion with severe pain decreased from one hundred percent to thirty-five percent. This reflects a substantial change in the day to day experience of patients who had been living with persistent severe pain [1].

Equally important is the reduction in fibromyalgia flares. The frequency of flares decreased by approximately 50 percent during the course of treatment, a finding that deserves particular emphasis. Flares are among the most disruptive features of fibromyalgia, unpredictable in their timing and often severe enough to prevent patients from maintaining a normal daily routine. A treatment that reduces their frequency by half does not simply lower a symptom score but changes the patient's ability to plan daily life, work, and maintain relationships. Together with the improvements in sleep, tender points, and everyday functioning reported by all twenty patients, this reflects a broad clinical benefit that goes beyond what is seen with analgesic or antidepressant treatment in this population [1].

The absence of adverse events in all twenty patients is an important finding, especially as safety concerns are often raised with less conventional therapies, yet in this study major autohemotherapy showed a safety profile that compares well with the pharmacological treatments commonly used in fibromyalgia. The fact that patients with a mean age of 50 years, equal numbers of men and women, and two years of established disease all completed the full treatment course without a single adverse event is consistent with the safety record of ozone therapy in the wider clinical literature and strengthens the case for its consideration in standard clinical practice [1].

What makes these results particularly meaningful is that pain reduction was not the only change observed. A treatment that acts on oxidative stress, inflammatory cytokines, mitochondrial function, erythrocyte deformability, and autonomic regulation at the same time does not produce improvement in one symptom while leaving the others unchanged. It shifts the overall biological state of the patient and that shift manifests across the full breadth of the condition's symptom profile. This is what distinguishes major autohemotherapy from the pharmacological options available to patients with fibromyalgia, not that it works better in a single domain, but that it acts across multiple domains at the same time and addresses the complexity of the condition rather than bypassing it [1].

Related Findings

The findings of this study are part of a growing body of clinical evidence developed over the past decade. Understanding how they fit within this broader context strengthens their significance and the case for ozone therapy as a valid approach to fibromyalgia management. The most methodologically rigorous evidence comes from randomized controlled trials. A double-blind placebo-controlled study by Sucuoğlu and Soydaş found statistically significant reductions in pain intensity and Fibromyalgia Impact Questionnaire scores in the ozone group compared to a sham procedure, establishing that the improvements associated with major autohemotherapy are not simply a placebo response [2]. An earlier randomized controlled trial by Fahmy similarly demonstrated superior outcomes with ozone therapy compared to a control condition, with clinically significant improvements in both pain and functional status [3].

The consistency of findings across larger observational studies is equally reassuring. Tirelli and colleagues examined outcomes in two hundred fibromyalgia patients treated with oxygen-ozone autohemotherapy and found clinically meaningful pain reductions in the majority, demonstrating that the effects observed in controlled settings translate reliably to the diversity of real-world clinical populations [4]. More recent retrospective analyses have added further depth to this picture. Çiftci İnceoğlu and colleagues reported significant reductions in pain, fatigue, and sleep disturbances with a favorable safety profile following major ozone autohemotherapy in fibromyalgia patients [5]. Also, Üşen and colleagues found that improvements in Fibromyalgia Impact Questionnaire scores, pain, and fatigue were maintained at medium-term follow-up, suggesting that the benefits of the treatment persist beyond the active treatment period, a question that the present study was not designed to address, and for which this observation is therefore a particularly relevant complement [6].

Further evidence from Tertemiz and colleagues demonstrated significant improvements across pain, sleep quality, and quality of life measures, reinforcing the pattern of multidomain improvement that is such a consistent feature of the ozone therapy literature in this condition [7]. Studies by Kuculmez and by Saxena and colleagues similarly confirmed meaningful improvements in pain and functional status, adding to the geographic and institutional diversity of a body of evidence that now spans multiple countries and clinical settings [8,9]. Alternative administration routes have also been studied with encouraging results, as ozonated water enema led to significant improvements in a randomized double blind trial [10], and rectal insufflation used as an add on treatment showed beneficial effects on pain and sleep in an earlier pilot study [11]. Together, these investigations make a compelling case that the therapeutic benefits of ozone in fibromyalgia are a property of the therapy itself rather than of any particular administration route or study population.

The biomarker evidence that has accumulated alongside the clinical studies gives these findings additional scientific weight. A systematic review and meta-analysis of ozone therapy's effects on oxidative stress markers across chronic inflammatory diseases found consistent reductions in lipid peroxidation products and increases in antioxidant enzyme activity, providing evidence that ozone therapy produces biological changes in the systems known to be dysregulated in fibromyalgia [12]. A prospective randomized clinical trial in chronic musculoskeletal pain patients with abnormal mitochondrial redox state found improvements in mitochondrial function biomarkers alongside pain reduction, providing direct evidence that ozone therapy's metabolic effects translate into clinical benefit in conditions sharing pathological features with fibromyalgia [13]. A comprehensive review confirmed consistent reductions in interleukin 6 and tumor necrosis factor alpha following ozone treatment in musculoskeletal conditions, changes that are consistent with its anti inflammatory mechanisms [14]. The effects of ozone therapy on mitochondrial function in chronic disease have been examined in detail, showing that low dose ozone offers a clear way to address problems at the mitochondrial level, which are directly related to the energy metabolism disturbances seen in fibromyalgia. [15].

Research in musculoskeletal pain provides a broader context for these findings. Comprehensive reviews of ozone therapy in musculoskeletal medicine have concluded that it represents a promising therapeutic option across a range of chronic pain conditions [16,17]. A critical review of clinical trials of medical ozone in musculoskeletal pain control concluded that the available evidence supports its therapeutic potential across multiple indications [18]. In addition, the preliminary evidence that ozone therapy combined with duloxetine produces better outcomes than either intervention alone is consistent with a synergistic model in which ozone addresses the oxidative, inflammatory, and metabolic dimensions that pharmacological agents do not reach [19]. This combination approach deserves formal evaluation in future research.

Conclusions and Future Directions

Fibromyalgia has often been approached as if it were a simpler condition than it really is. Most treatments have focused on single pathways, mainly through drugs that target neurotransmitters or pain sensitivity, yet the results have not matched what patients actually need. Clinical guidelines have gradually moved toward a more combined approach, placing greater emphasis on non pharmacological treatments, which reflects the limits of medication alone [20]. What this study adds is the observation that a single intervention, major autohemotherapy with ozone, can lead to improvements across multiple aspects of the condition, without side effects that often comes with using several drugs at the same time.

However, the limitations of the present study should not be minimized. Twenty patients without a control group cannot establish the causal certainty that a large randomized trial provides. Follow up data were not available, so it remains unclear how long the improvements last, and measures such as tender points, flare frequency, and medication use were based on patient reports rather than structured assessment. This does not take away from the improvements seen across a typical fibromyalgia population, but it points to what needs to come next, including larger randomized studies with consistent protocols, adequate sample sizes, longer follow up, and the inclusion of biological measures. It is also important to understand which patients are more likely to respond, including factors such as baseline oxidative stress, disease duration, or prior treatment history influence the outcome.

The need for standardized treatment protocols is another point that emerges clearly from the evidence. The variability in ozone concentration, blood volume, session number, and treatment frequency across the existing literature makes direct comparison between studies difficult and limits conclusions about optimal parameters. The development and wider use of agreed guidelines would be an important step toward the consistency the field still needs [21]. Equally important is greater integration of ozone therapy training into the continuing education of pain medicine specialists, so that the therapy is available to patients through practitioners who understand its mechanisms and its application.

Taken together, the evidence presents a clear and consistent picture. The mechanistic understanding, the biomarker findings, the clinical studies from independent groups, and the results of the present study all point in the same direction. Ozone therapy acts through its effects on the underlying biology of fibromyalgia, as it influences oxidative balance, inflammatory processes, mitochondrial function, oxygen delivery and autonomic regulation. These biological effects are well documented and the clinical improvements reported by patients can be understood in relation to them. Major autohemotherapy with ozone is not a cure for fibromyalgia. However, it represents a biologically grounded and clinically supported option that can offer benefit, particularly in patients who have not responded to conventional treatments.

References

1. Dimou T. LP004 The role of autohemotherapy with ozone as an effective treatment for fibromyalgia. European Society of Regional Anaesthesia and Pain Therapy (ESRA) Annual Congress; 2024. DOI: 10.1136/rapm-2024-ESRA.589.

2. Sucuoğlu H, Soydaş N. Efficacy of ozone therapy as an add-on treatment in fibromyalgia: a randomized double-blind placebo-controlled study. Journal of Back and Musculoskeletal Rehabilitation. 2023;36(2):357-66.

3. Tirelli U, Franzini M, Valdenassi L, Pandolfi S, Taibi R, Chirumbolo S. Fibromyalgia treated with oxygen-ozone auto-haemotherapy (O2-O3-AHT): a case study on 200 patients with a modified 10-PI-NRS evaluation. European Review for Medical and Pharmacological Sciences. 2022;26(21).

4. Fahmy Z. Controlled study of the efficacy ozone therapy in fibromyalgia, a randomised controlled trial. Journal of Ozone Therapy. 2019;3(4):20.

5. Çiftci İnceoğlu S, Ayyıldız A, Erden MF, Asik M, İnceoğlu A, Kuran B. Effects of major ozone autohemotherapy on fibromyalgia: a retrospective clinical study. Egyptian Rheumatology and Rehabilitation. 2026;53(1):16.

6. Üşen A, Özcan DS, Agirman M, Güner H, Kocyigit BF. Short- and medium-term effects of major ozone therapy on disease parameters in fibromyalgia syndrome: a retrospective study. Rheumatology International. 2025;45(4):72.

7. Tertemiz OF, Ozduran E, Gursoy S, Hanci V, Kaygusuz K, Ozbek IC, Sabuncu U. Effect of major ozone autohemotherapy in fibromyalgia syndrome: a retrospective study. PeerJ. 2025;13:e20475.

8. Kuculmez O. Effect of ozone therapy on pain and functional status in fibromyalgia patients. Alternative Therapies in Health and Medicine. 2025;31(1):10-14.

9. Saxena P, Komarraju S, Sathyanath D, Muralidharan S. Evaluating the efficacy of ozone therapy in fibromyalgia. Annals of African Medicine. 2026;10-4103.

10. Hou Q, Zhang J, Su Z, Wang X, Fang H, Qian S, Liao L. Clinical trial of ozonated water enema for the treatment of fibromyalgia: a randomized, double-blind trial. Pain Physician. 2025;28(1):E13.

11. Hidalgo-Tallón J, Menéndez-Cepero S, Vilchez JS, Rodríguez-López CM, Calandre EP. Ozone therapy as add-on treatment in fibromyalgia management by

rectal insufflation: an open-label pilot study. The Journal of Alternative and Complementary Medicine. 2013;19(3):238-42.

12. Alimohammadi M, Khoshnazar SM, Khajehpour H, Izadi M, Einollahi B, Hushmandi K. Effect of ozone therapy on oxidative stress indices in chronic inflammatory diseases: a systematic review and meta-analysis of randomized clinical trials. Advances in Redox Research. 2025;100143.

13. Eldemrdash A, Tairy T, Sabry L, Aelmulla A, Kamel M, Yousry E. Efficacy of medical ozone for treatment of chronic musculoskeletal pain with abnormal mitochondrial redox state: prospective randomized clinical trial. Pain Physician. 2024;27(4):E371.

14. de Sire A, Marotta N, Ferrillo M, Agostini F, Sconza C, Lippi L, Ammendolia A. Oxygen-ozone therapy for reducing pro-inflammatory cytokines serum levels in musculoskeletal and temporomandibular disorders: a comprehensive review. International Journal of Molecular Sciences. 2022;23(5):2528.

15. Viebahn-Haensler R, León Fernández OS. Mitochondrial dysfunction, its oxidative stress-induced pathologies and redox bioregulation through low-dose medical ozone: a systematic review. Molecules. 2024;29(12):2738.

16. Jeyaraman M, Jeyaraman N, Ramasubramanian S, Balaji S, Nallakumarasamy A, Patro BP, Migliorini F. Ozone therapy in musculoskeletal medicine: a comprehensive review. European Journal of Medical Research. 2024;29(1):398.

17. Serra ME, Baeza-Noci J, Mendes Abdala CV, Luvisotto MM, Bertol CD, Anzolin AP. The role of ozone treatment as integrative medicine. An evidence and gap map. Frontiers in Public Health. 2023;10:1112296.

18. de Araújo LT, da Silva PC, Masini M. Medical ozone as a therapeutic option in musculoskeletal pain control: a critical review of clinical trials considering safety and quality indicators for procedures and devices. The Yale Journal of Biology and Medicine. 2024;97(3):383.

19. Chen X, Zhou L, Mu J, Lu J, Xie J, Wang X, Ai C. Therapeutic effect of duloxetine combined with ozone trigger point injection on fibromyalgia: a retrospective observational study. 2021.

20. Macfarlane GJ, Kronisch C, Dean LE, Atzeni F, Häuser W, Fluss E, Choy E, Kosek E, Amris K, Branco J, Dincer FI. EULAR revised recommendations for the

management of fibromyalgia. Annals of the Rheumatic Diseases. 2017;76(2):318-28.

21. Konrad H. International Scientific Committee of Ozone Therapy ISCO3. 2014.

www.ingramcontent.com/pod-product-compliance
Lightning Source LLC
LaVergne TN
LVHW051131210926
848482LV00001B/57